Revitalized Radiance: Navigating the Empty Nest with Health and Happiness

Farewell Familiar Chaos

As the last echoes of bustling family life fade, Sarah, once the commander of a lively household, is faced with a newfound quiet. The empty nest syndrome sets in, and along with the emotional waves, unexpected challenges emerge. As the last echoes of laughter and footsteps fade away, Sarah finds herself standing in the doorway of an empty nest, a space that was once filled with the vibrant chaos of a bustling family. The quietude that settles in is both poignant and unfamiliar, and she takes a moment to absorb the profound change that has swept through her life.

The challenges ahead are as vast as the love she poured into raising her children, and yet, amidst the uncertainty, a journey of rediscovery unfolds.

For years, Sarah's identity was intricately woven into the roles of motherhood. From the early morning school runs to the chaotic family dinners, her life revolved around the needs and joys of her children. Now, with the rooms echoing emptiness and the once animated spaces silent, she faces the challenge of redefining herself outside the familiar confines of motherhood.

The first challenge is acknowledging the void left by the departure of her children. The empty rooms may symbolize physical absence, but the memories linger in every corner. Sarah grapples with the bittersweet truth that her children are spreading their wings and forging their own paths. Yet, amidst the ache of separation, she finds solace in the memories that fill the walls and a deep-seated pride in the independent individuals her children have become.

The second challenge is finding purpose beyond the roles of caretaker and nurturer. With the demands of motherhood diminishing, Sarah rediscovers her own passions and interests that were momentarily set aside. The empty nest becomes a canvas for her to paint new dreams and pursue neglected ambitions. Through this process, she learns that her identity extends beyond being a mother; it encompasses a tapestry of talents, dreams, and desires waiting to be explored.

Loneliness may loom as a formidable challenge, but Sarah soon discovers that the empty nest is an opportunity for rekindling connections. The relationship with her partner undergoes a renaissance as they navigate this new chapter together. With the children's absence, the focus shifts towards rediscovering the foundation of their companionship and creating a space for shared interests and adventures.

With the children now carving their own paths, the empty nest becomes both a literal and metaphorical space. The absence of daily familial demands allows her the freedom to reconsider long-standing habits, offering a canvas on which to paint the next chapter of her life. This introspective period becomes the foundation for a transformative journey, one where she seeks to rediscover herself amidst the newfound tranquility.

In the silence, she grapples with the echoes of old routines and ponders the meaning of self-care. The realization dawns that the bustling energy of family life had, in some ways, masked the importance of her own well-being. The quietude becomes a canvas upon which she sketches a vision of health and happiness, setting the stage for the challenges and triumphs that lie ahead. This chapter sets the tone for her journey towards revitalization, revealing that sometimes, the quietest moments speak the loudest.

Chapter 2: The Temptation Tango: Dancing with Delicious Dilemmas

Having bid farewell to the daily hustle of raising her family, Sarah found herself in an empty nest with newfound freedom. Sarah now well into her post-empty nest saga, she finds herself entangled in a comedic dance with the temptations of convenience and indulgence. Gone are the days of meal planning for a bustling household; now, it's just her and the siren call of the nearest drive-thru. Eager to explore the modern conveniences of technology, she stumbled upon the magical world of Uber Eats.

Sarah, once a maestro of meal planning, now reveled in the prospect of a carefree dining experience. Her smartphone became a portal to a plethora of culinary delights, offering everything from exotic cuisines to classic comfort foods. The possibilities were overwhelming, and for a moment, Sarah felt like a child in a digital candy store.

Opting for a Thai restaurant, she placed an order fit for royalty, and as she clicked 'confirm,' a sense of liberation washed over her. No more grocery lists, no more debating over chicken or fish— just a few taps on her phone, and dinner would be delivered to her doorstep.

Yet, as the delivery time approached, Sarah faced an unexpected dilemma. In the absence of meal planning, she realized she had nothing to fill her evenings. The once bustling kitchen, now silent in protest, challenged her to find new activities. Painting? Too messy. Knitting? Not thrilling enough. After much contemplation, she settled on learning to play the ukulele.

With the Thai food arriving, she strummed away on her newfound instrument, singing a comical tune about her liberation from the shackles of meal planning. Sarah's journey into the world of Uber Eats became a nightly adventure, each evening bringing a new culinary escapade. Her kitchen transformed into a haven for ukulele serenades, and she reveled in the freedom from the minutiae of meal planning.

In the midst of laughter, Thai food, and ukulele chords, Sarah embraced the joy of an empty nest. She relished the simple pleasures of spontaneity and the delicious convenience of a world at her fingertips—one Uber Eats order at a time.

The allure of late-night snacks and decadent treats sneaks in, whispering sweet promises of instant gratification. The pantry, once stocked with family-sized boxes of crackers and cookies, now seems to echo with the laughter of mischievous snacks daring her to break free from the constraints of health-conscious choices.

Balancing cravings with nourishment become a theatrical performance, a culinary ballet that plays out in her kitchen. She contemplates the intricate choreography of choosing a salad over a pizza, realizing that the delicate dance between temptation and discipline requires a fine-tuned sense of humor and a healthy dose of self-love.

Through laughter and a touch of self-deprecating humor, she embraces the fact that sometimes, life's delicate dance involves a shimmy between a salad fork and a chocolate truffle.

Chapter 3: Dancing Spoons and Culinary Capers: Kitchen Adventures for One

Sarah becomes aware of the pitfalls of her post-parental saga and her new close relationship with food delivery, a remarkable transformation takes place in the heart of her home—the kitchen. What was once a utilitarian space for whipping up family feasts becomes her very own stage, and the dance of spatulas, pans, and pots unfolds in a hilarious culinary symphony. It's a one-woman show, and Sarah is ready to rock the apron.

The journey commences with a recipe book so thick it could double as a doorstop, filled with ingredients that sound like they've taken a detour from a foreign language immersion class.

Undaunted, Sarah, now a self-proclaimed culinary maestro, dons a chef's hat—figuratively, of course, because let's be honest, hats in the kitchen are more for show than anything else. Armed with newfound kitchen bravado, she bravely faces the spice rack, wondering if cumin and coriander will ever reconcile their differences in her kitchen tango.

Enter the era of experimentation, where the kitchen witnesses a series of flavorful fiascos that could give any cooking show blooper reel a run for its money. From mistaking salt for sugar to attempting a daring dance with a hot chili pepper, our fearless solo chef navigates the challenges with the grace of a ballerina and the comedic timing of a stand-up comedian. The kitchen becomes her stage, and every mishap is a punchline in this culinary comedy.

Armed with newfound enthusiasm and a recipe she found online titled "Gourmet Delights for the Brave Soul," Sarah embarked on a journey that would soon become the stuff of kitchen legends.

The recipe called for exotic ingredients like truffle oil, saffron threads, and a rare spice known as "dragon tears" (which, unbeknownst to Sarah, was just a fancy name for extra-hot chili powder). Undeterred by the seemingly unpronounceable items on the list, she donned her imaginary chef's hat and decided to channel her inner culinary goddess.

As Sarah joyfully minced and chopped her way through the ingredients, she couldn't help but feel a sense of accomplishment. Little did she know that her kitchen was about to transform into a stage for a culinary catastrophe of epic proportions.

The first sign that things were veering off course came when she misread "1 teaspoon of salt" as "1 tablespoon of salt." The unsuspecting pot bubbled away with an ocean's worth of saltiness. Undeterred, Sarah soldiered on, determined to salvage her gourmet creation.

Next up was the saffron, a spice she had never encountered before. In her attempt to be generous with the golden threads, she mistook the saffron container for the pepper shaker. The dish now had a vibrant orange hue reminiscent of a sunset, but the taste was more like a fiery sunrise.

The pièce de résistance was the truffle oil, a luxurious ingredient that Sarah had splurged on for this special occasion. Eagerly drizzling it into the pot, she soon discovered that truffle oil, when used with a heavy hand, can turn a dish from gourmet to greasy disaster. Her kitchen, once filled with the promise of culinary glory, now smelled like a confused mix of a French bistro and a fast-food joint.

As she took her first hesitant bite, Sarah's taste buds went on a rollercoaster ride of confusion. The dragon tears, the salt overload, and the overpowering truffle oil created a symphony of flavors that left her palate in a state of shock. She pondered whether her taste buds had signed up for a culinary boot camp without her consent.

In the end, Sarah's "Gourmet Delights for the Brave Soul" turned out to be a lesson in humility and a testament to the resilience of the human spirit. As she sat amidst the remnants of her culinary experiment, Sarah couldn't help but burst into laughter. The kitchen, now a battlefield of mismatched ingredients, had become the stage for a comedy of culinary errors.

And so, with a heart full of laughter and a slightly singed sense of taste, Sarah learned that not every recipe is meant to be conquered. Sometimes, the greatest culinary adventures are the ones that teach you to appreciate the simplicity of a well-cooked egg or the comforting embrace of a familiar spaghetti Bolognese. In the kitchen of life, even a culinary disaster can be a recipe for laughter and a delicious reminder that not every journey needs a gourmet ending.

Despite the occasional culinary catastrophe, the joy of cooking for one begins to radiate. The sizzling pans create a kitchen orchestra, and the aroma of spices fills the air like a symphony of flavors. Our solo chef discovers that healthy eating is not just about the destination; it's the delightful journey of experimenting with new flavors, even if those flavors occasionally come with a side of unexpected spice-induced tears. So here's to our empty nest chef, turning culinary chaos into comedic gold, one kitchen dance at a time. Bon appétit and a hearty chuckle!

Chapter 4: A Comedic Exercise in Fitness

Now that he aroma of home-cooked meals wafted through the air, Sarah, having indulged in her culinary pursuits a bit too enthusiastically found herself facing a pair of jeans that seemed to have suddenly shrunk. It was a classic case of too much love for her own cooking, and the evidence was snugly wrapped around her midsection.

Determined to face the expanding situation head-on, Sarah decided it was time to introduce a new character into her life — Exercise. Armed with a yoga mat, a water bottle, and an unbridled enthusiasm that was almost alarming, she embarked on a fitness journey that promised to be both entertaining and slightly awkward.

Her first venture into the world of home workouts was a YouTube video titled "Dance Your Way to Fitness with Zumba Zara." Sarah, with the grace of a misplaced giraffe, attempted to mirror Zara's fancy footwork. What started as a dance quickly turned into a comedic interpretation of interpretative dance, with limbs flailing in unexpected directions. The living room witnessed an unexpected performance as Sarah jived, shuffled, and occasionally tripped over her own enthusiasm.

Next up was the world of cardio, where Sarah discovered the joys of high-intensity interval training. Bursting with energy, she sprinted in place like a determined jackrabbit, blissfully unaware of her cat observing from the couch with a mix of curiosity and mild concern. Halfway through, Sarah decided to throw in a couple of jumping jacks, transforming her living room into a makeshift trampoline park.

Yoga, the supposed Zen oasis of exercise, proved to be the greatest challenge. Sarah contorted herself into positions that seemed to defy the laws of physics. The downward dog became the "confused cat," and the warrior pose resembled more of a "flustered flamingo." At one point, she accidentally knocked over a potted plant, turning her downward dog into an impromptu gardening session.

After a week of Sarah's energetic attempts at fitness, her living room resembled a battlefield of misplaced enthusiasm. The cat had taken refuge on top of the fridge, and the potted plant had found a new home on the windowsill. Yet, amidst the chaos, something magical happened – Sarah found herself laughing.

She realized that exercise wasn't just about shedding pounds; it was an adventure of its own, a comedy show starring an unlikely fitness enthusiast. Sarah's living room became a stage where laughter was the cardio, and her attempts at exercise were the highlight reel.

In the end, as Sarah caught her breath amidst the disheveled living room, she realized that the journey to a healthier lifestyle didn't have to be a serious affair. It could be a joyous, laughter-filled romp through the world of jumping jacks, interpretive dance, and bewildered yoga poses. And so, armed with a newfound appreciation for the comedic side of fitness, Sarah embraced the delightful chaos of her exercise routine, confident that, in the grand theater of life, a good laugh is the best exercise of all.

Chapter 5: Craving Comfort: Navigating the Emotional Eating Maze

In the quiet echoes of solitude and falling off the exercise roller coaster Sarah realises the emotions attached to her relationship with food; revealing a poignant journey through the emotional labyrinth that influences her eating habits. The refrigerator, once a mere appliance, now stands as a fortress of comfort in moments of vulnerability, as the battle between emotions and nourishment becomes a heart-wrenching odyssey, or as Sarah fondly calls it, "The Refrigerator Chronicles: A Love-Hate Affair."

As Sarah grapples with the quiet spaces left by departed laughter and the tangible absence of familial chaos, emotions bubble to the surface like a simmering pot of emotional soup. Loneliness, nostalgia, and even the echoes of unspoken dreams find solace in the pantry's embrace. In these moments, food becomes both a shield and a sword, offering fleeting comfort while silently waging war on the spirit within.

In confronting her emotional eating tendencies, Sarah embarks on a quest to understand the complexity of her relationship with food. The chocolate bars in the pantry whisper promises of sweetness, and the salty chips extend an invitation to a temporary escape from the solitude. Yet, in the midst of this emotional turbulence, she discovers an inner strength to explore alternative coping mechanisms.

As Sarah embarks on her culinary odyssey, armed with nothing but a spoon and a well-worn spatula, she discovers that each bite is like a tiny, edible time machine. The taste of chocolate chip cookies catapults her back to family bake-offs, where flour fights were inevitable, and victory tasted oh-so-sweet. A forkful of mac and cheese becomes a cheesy embrace, reminiscent of lazy Sunday afternoons with her kids. With every mouthful, she unearths the raw vulnerability beneath her cravings, realizing that her emotional palate is as diverse as a buffet at an indecisive eater's dream wedding.

In this gastronomic journey, Sarah begins to rewrite the narrative of her relationship with food. The once-dreaded salad now becomes a superhero, swooping in to save the day when guilt about yesterday's pizza threatens to overwhelm her. She even contemplates a romantic comedy starring her and a bowl of kale as they navigate the tumultuous world of self-discovery and leafy greens. Each morsel becomes a pen in her culinary diary, jotting down tales of love, laughter, and the occasional wrestling match with a stubborn pickle jar. As she munches her way through the buffet of emotions, Sarah realizes that the key to a happy tummy is not just in the flavors on the plate but in the memories and longings that each taste brings to the table. And so, armed with newfound wisdom and maybe a spoonful of ice cream for good measure, she continues to savor the comedy that is life—one bite at a time.

In a plot twist worthy of a Hollywood script, Sarah embraces a healthier connection with nourishment. She explores mindfulness, meditation, and journaling as outlets for emotional expression. The quiet moments, once filled with the clatter of family life, now become opportunities for introspection and healing. Through a journey of self-compassion, Sarah finds the courage to navigate the emotional eating maze and emerges on the other side with a heartwarming understanding of herself and a newfound appreciation for the nourishment that extends beyond the plate.

The refrigerator, once a crutch, becomes a symbol of resilience, a source of sustenance, and a reminder that, even in solitude, one can find solace in the nourishment of the heart. Sarah's love-hate affair with emotional eating transforms into a heartwarming tale of self-discovery, proving that the refrigerator may house more than just leftovers—it can also be a repository of courage, healing, and the occasional pint of ice cream.

Chapter 6: Cheers to Accountability: The Accountability Allies Comedy Club

Sarah found herself at a crossroads. Staring into the mirror one morning, she decided it was time for a change – a commitment to wellness. But Sarah, being a woman of creativity and flair, didn't opt for the conventional gym or a strict diet. Instead, she turned her pursuit of accountability into a lively comedy club.

Armed with a newfound determination, Sarah donned a metaphorical cape and embarked on a quest to recruit the most reliable sidekicks in the accountability business. The first stop? The family WhatsApp group.

What was once a platform for mundane discussions about weekend plans and grocery lists transformed into a lively arena of wellness updates. Sarah shamelessly shared her latest yoga poses, salad creations, and, of course, the occasional indulgence. The family chat turned into a virtual stand-up comedy show where healthy habits took center stage, and laughter echoed through the digital space.

It all started when Sarah decided to turn her pursuit of wellness into a side-splitting adventure, and the focal point was none other than the family WhatsApp group.

In the midst of usual discussions about what to have for dinner and whose turn it was to take out the trash, Sarah boldly stepped into the limelight. Armed with a kale smoothie in one hand and a yoga mat in the other, she announced her grand entrance into the world of wellness.

"Guess what, everyone! I've officially become a yoga master and a salad enthusiast," Sarah declared, attaching a photo of herself contorted into a seemingly impossible pose with a plate of greens in the background.

Cue the entrance of her family, bewildered and amused by the unexpected twist in their daily digital banter. Her brother responded with a meme featuring a confused cat attempting a downward dog, and her mom chimed in, "Honey, are you sure that's not just a pretzel?"

Undeterred by the teasing, Sarah turned the family chat into a virtual comedy club, and her wellness escapades became the star attraction. Gym mishaps were the first chapter in this hilarity-filled saga. Sarah shared a story about attempting a new workout routine that involved an enthusiastic jump onto a treadmill—only to discover it wasn't moving. "Who knew treadmills could be so sneaky?" she quipped.

The accidental kale smoothie disasters became a recurring theme in the sitcom of her wellness journey. Sarah's attempt at creating a superfood elixir resulted in a concoction so green it could've been mistaken for paint. Her friends suggested it looked like something Shrek would drink, and the nickname "Shrek Shake" became an instant hit in the group.

Then there were the collective groans over leg day. Sarah, always the enthusiast, shared a video of herself attempting a set of lunges, only to lose her balance and topple over. Her friend jokingly commented, "I think your legs just declared independence."

As the weeks passed, the family WhatsApp group transformed into a stage for laughter, with Sarah as the fearless comedian narrating her wellness misadventures. The more absurd the workout, the funnier the story. Laughter truly became the ultimate medicine, and the family eagerly awaited the daily dosage of comedic relief.

Even when setbacks occurred, like Sarah's accidental mid-week ice cream binge, the group rallied together with supportive emojis and gifs. "Well, they say laughter burns calories, right?" Sarah defended herself.

The sitcom of wellness continued to unfold, with each shared victory and mishap adding another punchline to the script. As the laughter echoed through the digital space, it became clear that in the world of Sarah's wellness journey, humor was the best workout partner anyone could ask for. And so, the family WhatsApp group became not just a source of connection but a hub of laughter and joy, all thanks to Sarah's hilarious take on the pursuit of health.

Online communities became the digital stage where the Accountability Allies gathered. Memes, recipes, and the occasional "Can someone please motivate me to put on workout clothes?" cry for help filled the virtual space. The camaraderie built through shared experiences turned the quest for accountability into a joyous festival of encouragement and laughter.

Through the laughter and lighthearted banter, our empty nest mother discovered the power of accountability allies. They became the backbone of her wellness journey, cheering her on in moments of triumph and offering a virtual shoulder to lean on during inevitable setbacks. The comedy club of accountability not only transformed the pursuit of health into a delightful adventure but also underscored the profound impact of shared laughter and support on the road to wellness.

And so, the Accountability Allies Comedy Club became a symbol of unity, laughter, and the unexpected joy found in the pursuit of wellness. As Sarah continued her journey, she realized that, indeed, wellness could be both amusing and deeply fulfilling. Cheers to the Accountability Allies Comedy Club!

Chapter 7: Joyful Journeys and Non-Scale Triumphs

Sarah undergoes a profound shift in perspective, turning her wellness journey into a celebration of non-scale victories. With a twirl and a skip, she sidesteps the often-intimidating bathroom scale, choosing instead to revel in the tangible benefits that extend far beyond mere numbers.

Her day began with an ode to increased energy, a lyrical celebration that unfolded with the rising sun. It was the kind of energy that made Sarah bounce out of bed, her feet barely touching the floor as she embraced the morning with a vitality that transcended any numeric representation. No longer enslaved by the fluctuating needle on the scale,

Sarah had discovered a different metric for success—one measured in the effortless spring in her step and the boundless enthusiasm that accompanied her every move.

As the sun streamed through her bedroom window, casting a warm glow on the walls, Sarah marveled at the transformation taking place within her. She had embarked on a journey not to fit into a certain dress size or achieve an arbitrary number on the scale, but rather to reclaim a sense of joy and energy that had long eluded her.

Her morning routine became a dance of vitality—a symphony of stretches, deep breaths, and moments of gratitude for the body that carried her through each day. The mirror, once a source of self-critique, now reflected the glow of newfound confidence and an unspoken promise to embrace life with open arms.

People noticed the change in Sarah. The local bakery owner, who used to see her reluctantly eyeing the calorie counts on the pastries, now witnessed her selecting a treat with a smile, savoring the indulgence without a hint of guilt. The park regulars observed a woman jogging with a lightness in her step, her laughter echoing through the air.

Sarah's success was no longer quantified by numbers on a scale but manifested in the vibrancy she brought to every aspect of her life. She joined a local dance class, not to burn calories, but to revel in the joy of movement. The once-dreaded gym became a playground where she explored the capabilities of her body, discovering strength and agility she never knew she possessed.

Her friends noticed the change too, not just in her appearance, but in the way she approached life with a newfound zest. The chapter of increased energy became a story of transformation—one that radiated from the inside out. Sarah's vitality became contagious, inspiring those around her to redefine their own measures of success.

Sarah relished in the simplicity of feeling alive. No longer burdened by the expectations of a scale, she measured her success in the genuine smiles, the genuine laughter, and the genuine moments of joy that marked her journey. Her community became witness to a woman who had unlocked the secret to true vitality—one that couldn't be confined to any numeric representation but rather one that danced freely with the rhythm of her heart.

The scale, once a feared judge, now takes a backseat to the spotlight on improved mood. Laughter becomes the soundtrack of her days, a melody that echoes through the once-silent hallways of the empty nest. The joy of making healthier choices resonates not just in the meals she prepares but in the newfound lightness that permeates her spirit.

Tangible benefits unfold like petals of a flourishing flower. The glow of her skin, the clarity of her mind, and the strength in her body become markers of triumph. No longer defined by pounds and ounces, she revels in the non-scale victories that paint her wellness journey in hues of vibrant well-being.

Celebrating these victories becomes a daily ritual—an affirmation of the positive changes that ripple through her life. Whether it's effortlessly lifting grocery bags, feeling the strength in a morning stretch, or delighting in the compliments that hint at her radiant transformation, each non-scale triumph becomes a trophy on the mantle of her wellness adventure.

Sarah has learned that the true measure of success is not confined to a numerical scale but is found in the joyous journey of increased energy, improved mood, and the tangible benefits that grace her every step. With every celebration, she takes a bow, recognizing that the real victory lies not in the pounds shed but, in the happiness, gained; a testament to the transformative power of embracing and savoring the non-scale victories that make every step of the journey worthwhile.

Chapter 8: Radiant Revelations: A Heartfelt Farewell to the Nest

In the grand finale of Sarah's radiance, unfolds as a heartwarming symphony of reflections, gratitude, and the sheer bliss of radiant well-being. With a sigh of contentment, she embraces the season of change, recognizing that her journey is not just about adapting to an empty nest but about cultivating a life brimming with health, happiness, and an enduring vitality.

As she pens the final chapter, she gazes back at the laughter, tears, and the comedic escapades that have woven the tapestry of her wellness adventure. The journey, once a series of challenges, becomes a cherished narrative of self-discovery, resilience, and the delightful surprises that come with embracing change.

The empty nest, once a symbol of solitude, now becomes a canvas painted with the vibrant hues of her newfound health. The kitchen, once a place of solitude, transforms into a culinary haven where nourishment is not just about sustenance, but an art form celebrated with every colorful ingredient.

She reflects on the treadmill escapades, the Zumba zest, and the outdoor outtakes with a smile, realizing that the journey to fitness is not just about the destination but the joyous exploration of movement that brings laughter and vitality.

The emotional eating maze, once a labyrinth of cravings, becomes a testament to her resilience and the discovery of healthier coping mechanisms. The refrigerator, once a crutch, stands as a symbol of nourishment—of the body, mind, and spirit.

The quest for accountability, once a virtual comedy club, becomes a testament to the power of shared laughter and support in fostering lasting lifestyle changes. The scale, once a daunting judge, steps aside to make room for the celebration of non-scale victories that radiate health, happiness, and an infectious vibrancy.

As our empty nest mother basks in the glow of her radiant revelations, she realizes that the journey was not just about adapting to an empty nest but about transforming it into a sanctuary of well-being. The season of change becomes a dance of gratitude, as she acknowledges the beauty in each twist and turn, the highs and lows, and the laughter and tears that have shaped her into the vibrant, resilient, and joy-filled person she is today.

And so, with a heart full of gratitude, a spirit ablaze with vitality, and a radiant smile that mirrors the beauty of her journey, our protagonist bids a heartfelt farewell to the nest. She steps into the next season of life with newfound health, happiness, and an everlasting appreciation for the transformative power of embracing change.

Closing- Call to health and peace

As the final chapter unfolds, it's not just a farewell; it's a spirited invitation for each reader to relish their personal season of transformation. Let it be a call to embark on a profound journey towards a radiant and fulfilling life. Sarah's story teaches us that the pursuit of health and well-being is not confined to numbers on a scale but is a vibrant dance of embracing vitality, joy, and self-discovery. Like a beacon, it beckons us all to step into our own narratives, to rewrite our chapters with enthusiasm and resilience. So, seize the invitation with open arms, savor the moments of change, and let your journey towards well-being be a radiant celebration of the beautiful, transformative seasons that await. Embrace the power within you to redefine success, and may your path be adorned with the genuine smiles, laughter, and moments of joy that mark a truly fulfilling and healthy life.

Thank you,

Jennifer